Mediterranean Seafood Recipes

50 Unmissable Seafood Recipes for Your Mediterranean Diet

Alex Brawn

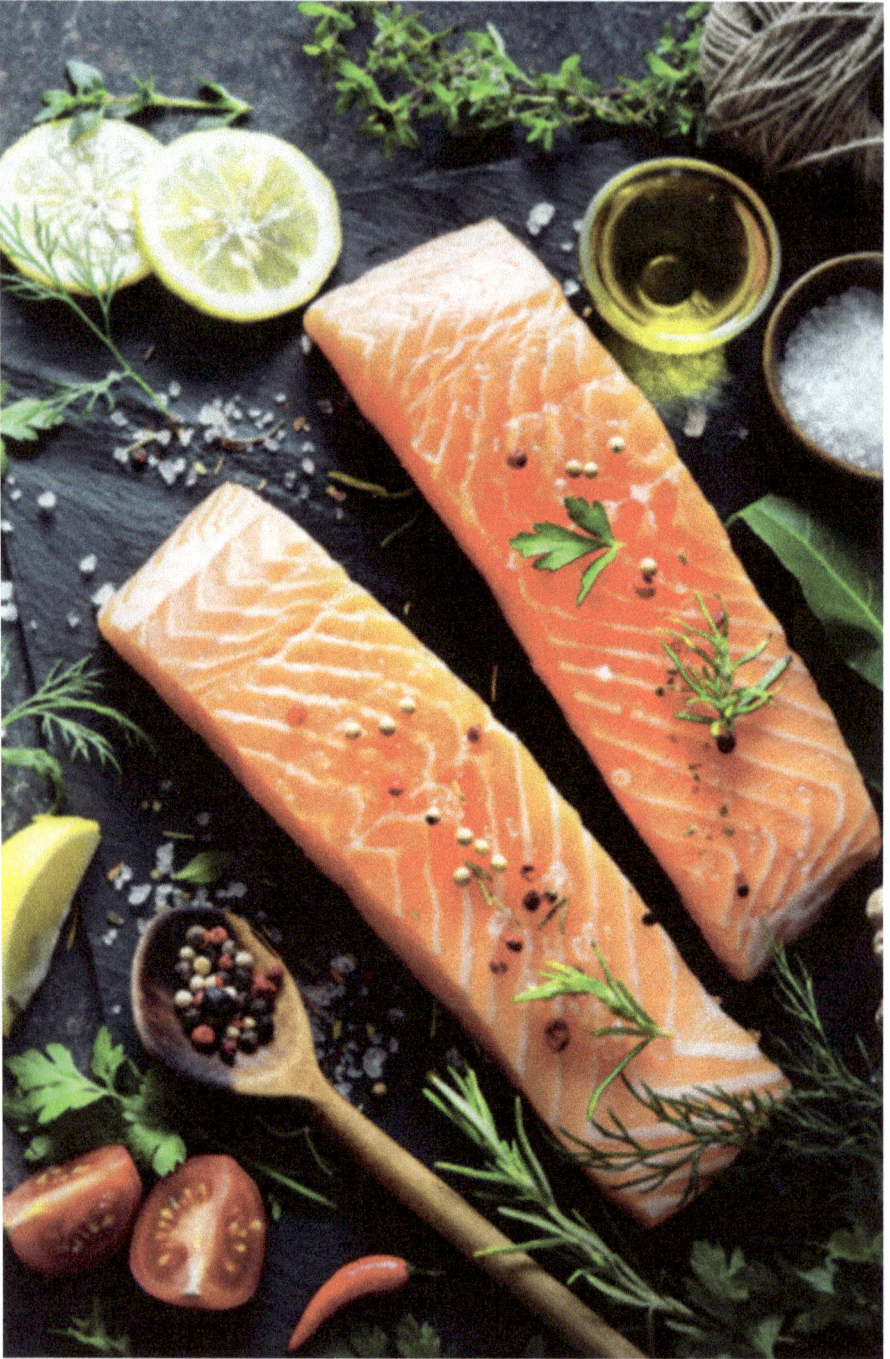

Table of Contents

Authentic aguachile with shrimp

This Mediterranean Sea diet recipe is simple, yet flavorful and tasty appetizer similar to ceviche recipe.

Ingredients

- 1 serrano chili, sliced in half lengthwise
- 1 teaspoon of kosher salt
- 2 large limes
- 1 cup of cilantro
- ½ cup of fresh lime juice
- Pinch of salt
- ¼ of a red onion, thinly sliced
- Splash of white vinegar
- 1 pound of raw shrimp
- Water
- 1 garlic clove
- 2 jalapeños, sliced in half lengthwise

Directions

- Place the sliced shrimp in a shallow serving dish in one layer.
- Squeeze lime to cover the shrimp, turning slightly pink.

- Sprinkle with a little salt.
- Cook the shrimp turning over as needed in the lime juice for 20 minutes.
- Season the red onion with salt.
- Pour just enough water to cover the onions, add a splash of white vinegar.
- Combine lime juice, cilantro, jalapeno, chili, and kosher salt in a food processor, blend till smooth.
- Pour the mixture over the shrimp and toss to coat.
- Drain the onions and scatter them over, mixing slightly.
- Refrigerate for 4 hours.
- Taste, and adjust accordingly.
- Serve and enjoy with tortilla chips.

Roasted mustard seed white fish with potato Brussel sprout hash

Ingredients

- 10 ounces of potatoes, thinly sliced
- 2 teaspoons of olive oil
- Salt and pepper to taste
- 1 large shallot, thinly sliced
- 1 tablespoon of olive oil
- 6 ounce filets of fish
- 4 teaspoons of whole grain mustard
- 8 ounces of Brussel Sprouts, thinly sliced
- Pinch of caraway seeds

Directions

- Firstly, preheat your oven ready to 450°F.
- Slice potatoes and shallots, toss with oil, salt and pepper in a mixing bowl.
- Place on a parchment lined baking sheet in a single layer, let bake for 20 minutes.
- Slice and place Brussel sprouts in the same oily bowl.

- Toss, then, add a pinch of caraway seeds . Set aside.
- Mix the whole grain mustard together with oil in a small bowl.
- Season the fish with salt and pepper.
- Divide the mustard mixture, then spoon over the fish.
- When the potatoes have baked for 20 minutes, add the brussel sprouts, toss.
- Make a spot for the fish, let bake for 12 minutes, until cooked through.
- Divide the potato Brussel sprout hash among two bowls and top with the mustard glazed fish.
- Serve and enjoy.

Pomegranate glazed mackerel with satsuma and fennel salad

Ingredients

- 4 mackerel fillets
- 40ml of runny honey
- 2 medium beetroots
- 1 tablespoon of pomegranate molasses
- 1 small red onion
- 1 teaspoon of runny honey
- 1 small fennel
- 40ml of pomegranate molasses
- 6 satsumas
- 1 bunch of fresh dill
- 4 tablespoons of extra virgin olive oil
- 1 lemon

Directions

- Preheat the oven ready to 400°F.
- Then, wrap each beetroot individually in foil, let roast for 45 minutes, let cool.

- In a large bowl, combine the pomegranate molasses together with the honey and 40ml of satsuma, season.
- Place the mackerel into the mixture, let marinate for 20 minutes.
- Combine sliced satsuma with the red onion, fennel and beetroot. Set aside.
- Also, combine the olive oil together with the lemon juice, molasses, and honey in a small bowl, whisk. Set aside for later.
- Remove the mackerel fillets from the marinade and place on a baking tray lined with foil.
- Transfer the marinade into a small saucepan, bring to the boil over a high heat for 5 minutes. Set aside for the glaze.
- Preheat your grill to high, grill the fillets for 4 minutes.
- Remove from the oven and brush with the glaze, then season.
- Drizzle the vinaigrette over the salad and toss to combine.

- Roughly chop and add the dill.
- Serve and enjoy with the mackerel.

Coconut lemongrass scallops with lime

The coconut lemongrass scallop recipe is stuffed with herbs and lime zest for a healthy Mediterranean Sea diet.

Ingredients

- 4 tablespoons of white vinegar
- 1 can of coconut milk
- Kaffir lime leaves
- 1 stalk of fresh lemongrass, smashed
- 1 large lime zest and juice
- 1 ½ teaspoons of fish sauce
- Slices red chili
- 1 ¼ pound of large scallops
- 1 tablespoon coconut oil
- 1 shallot, diced
- Salt and pepper
- 8 leaves of fresh basil
- 2 thin slices ginger

Directions

- Cook a small pot of rice on stove.

- In a small saucepan, simmer, on low heat, shallot in vinegar, until vinegar reduces in 5 minutes.
- Add coconut milk with smashed lemongrass, ½ of the lime zest, and ginger, let simmer on low heat for 5 minutes.
- Stir in fish sauce and lime juice.
- Taste, and adjust accordingly. Let rest and flavors infuse.
- Rinse, pat dry scallops.
- Then, season with salt and pepper.
- In a skillet, heat coconut oil over medium heat.
- When hot enough, add the scallops and sear each side for 3 minutes.
- Divide rice between bowls, top with scallops, place flavorful lemongrass coconut sauce over the top.
- Serve and enjoy.

Smoked salmon, avocado, and fennel salad

Ingredients

- 6 ounces of smoked salmon
- ⅓ cup of mayo
- 2 tablespoons capers
- 1/3 cup of sour cream
- 1 tablespoon of olive oil
- 1 avocado , sliced
- ¼ cup of thinly sliced red onion
- 2 tablespoons of lemon juice
- 2 garlic cloves-finely minced
- 1/3 cup of fresh dill, chopped
- Sunflower sprouts
- ¼ heaping teaspoon of salt
- ¼ teaspoon of fresh cracked pepper
- 1 head of butter lettuce
- 1 Turkish cucumber, sliced
- ½ a fennel bulb, thinly sliced

Directions

- Combine mayo, sour cream, olive oil, lemon juice, garlic, salt and pepper in a bowl, whisk until smooth.
- Add the dill, then mix. Set aside.
- Place the lettuce together with the fennel bulb, smoked salmon, cucumber, red onion, and capers in a big bowl.
- Toss, then add enough dressing to coat.
- Divide the salad and garnish with avocado and sprinkle with salt and pepper.
- Serve and enjoy.

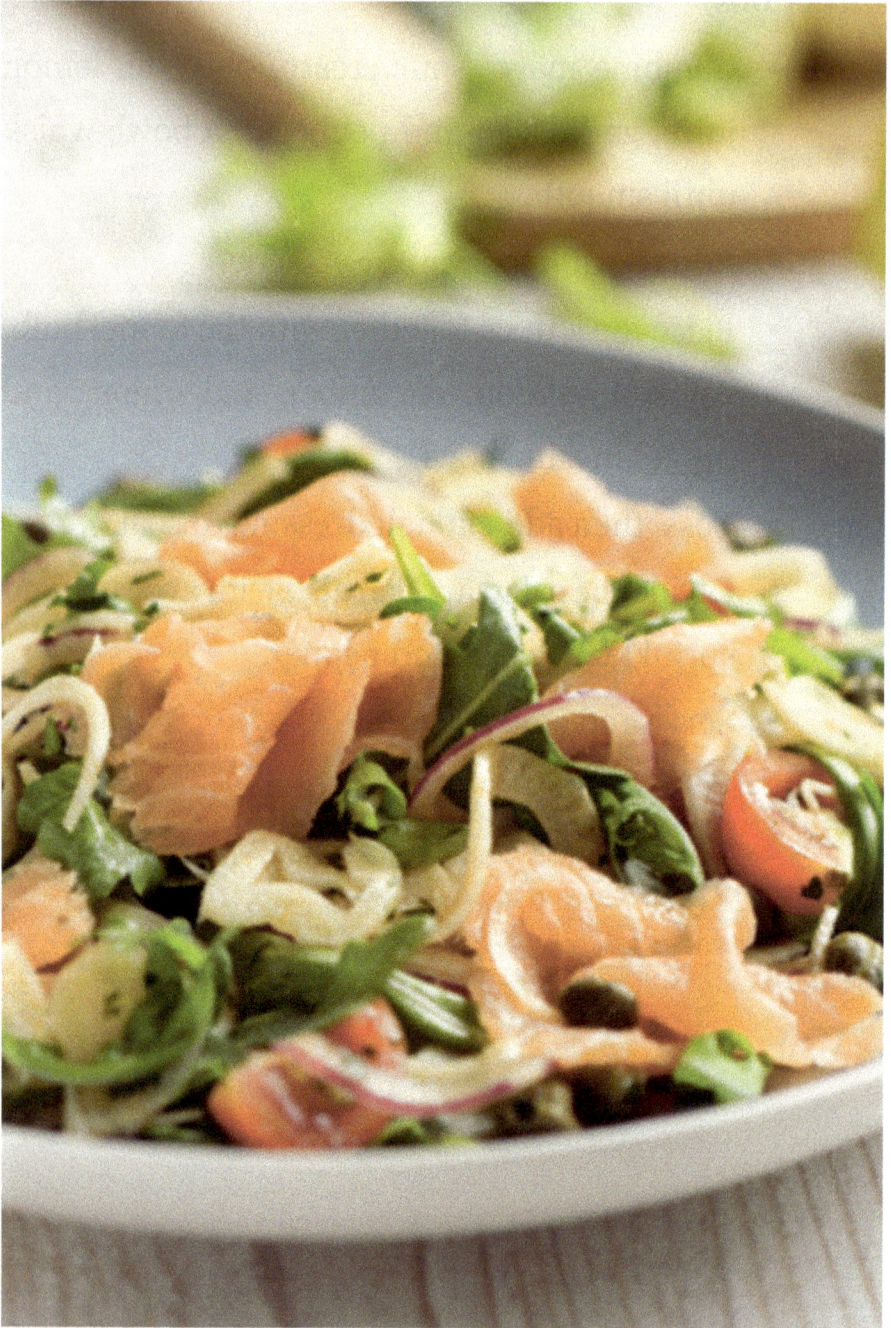

Dover sole with lemon, dill, and leeks

Ingredients

- 2 tablespoons of fresh dill, chopped
- 2 medium leeks, thinly sliced
- ⅛ teaspoon of kosher salt
- 10 ounces of dover sole
- 5teaspoons of olive oil
- 1 teaspoon of salt and pepper
- 8 ounces of baby potatoes
- 1 tablespoon of lemon juice
- Zest from ½ a lemon

Directions

- Place sliced potatoes and leeks in a medium bowl and toss with olive oil, pepper, salt, and lemon zest.
- Place on a parchment lined sheet-pan in a single layer in the oven.
- Let bake for 20 minutes, tossing.
- Add the fish to the same bowl, drizzle with oil, salt , pepper and remaining lemon zest.
- Toss to coat all sides. Keep aside.

- Combine dill, olive oil, lemon juice and kosher salt in a bowl.
- Lay the fish over top of ready potatoes and return to the oven.
- Let bake for 10 minutes.
- Serve and enjoy.

Smoked salmon hand rolls with avocado

Ingredients

- 3 cups of calrose rice
- 2 cups of sprouts
- 2 packages nori sheets
- 2 tablespoons of seasoned rice wine vinegar
- Wasabi paste
- 2 teaspoon of toasted sesame seeds
- 16 ounces of smoked salmon
- 8 ounces of sliced mushrooms
- Soy sauce
- 1 tablespoon of oil
- 1 teaspoon of soy sauce
- 1 red bell pepper
- 1 cucumber, cut into strips
- 2 avocados , cut into strips

Directions

- Bring rice to a boil, cover, and simmer on low for 20 minutes.
- Place rice in a wood bowl , sprinkle with the seasoned rice vinegar .

- Slice the rice and sprinkle with toasted sesame seeds and cover with a damp kitchen towel .

- Sauté mushrooms in olive oil over medium heat.

- Add sesame oil , cook for 2 more minutes.

- Season with soy sauce .

- Place bell pepper, cucumber and avocado in individual bowls.

- Place the sprouts in a bowl and smoked salmon on a small platter

- Place nori sheet horizontally.

- Spread sushi rice on the left half of the sheet, align strips of veggies, diagonally. top with smoked salmon, mushrooms, and sprouts.

- Serve and enjoy.

Baked cod recipe with garlic and lemon

Ingredients

- 3 tablespoon of olive oil
- 2 tablespoons of finely chopped preserved lemon
- 1 teaspoon of kosher salt
- ½ cup of white wine
- ½ teaspoon of pepper
- 1 large bunch asparagus
- Zest from 1 lemon
- 1 large fennel bulb
- Cod
- Pinch salt and pepper
- ½ cup of chicken
- 1 large leek, white
- 4 cloves garlic, rough chopped
- 2 teaspoons of fresh thyme
- 1 tablespoons of fresh thyme

Directions

- Preheat oven to 400°F.

- Place cod in a bowl, drizzle with olive oil and sprinkle with salt and pepper, thyme, and zest.
- Heat olive oil over medium heat.
- Add fennel, sauté for 7 minutes, stir.
- Add leeks and garlic, continue cooking, stirring.
- Add preserved lemon with the fresh thyme, broth, and white wine.
- Stir in salt and pepper and let simmer on low heat for 5 minutes.
- Nestle in the fish in the pan, bake for 10 minutes.
- Serve and enjoy.

White miso black cod

Ingredients

- 1/3 cup of sugar
- 3 tablespoons of sake
- 4 x 4 ounce pieces of Black Cod
- 1/3 cup of white miso paste
- 3 tablespoons of mirin

Directions

- Bring the mirin and sake to a boil.
- Whisk in the miso until dissolved.
- Add the sugar and cook over moderate heat, whisk.
- Transfer the marinade to a large baking dish and let cool
- Add the fish to the marinade and turn to coat.
- Refrigerate overnight.
- Preheat your oven ready to 400°F.
- Heat a small oil, the wipe the marinade off the fish.
- Place the fish, skin side up, in the skillet, sear until golden.

- Turnover, crisp up the skin for 3 minutes.
- Roast for 10 more minutes.
- Serve and enjoy.

Baked salmon recipe with asparagus and yogurt dill sauce

Ingredients

- 1 large bunch asparagus
- 1 ¼ lb. of wild king salmon filet
- 2 tablespoons [olive oil](#)
- Squeeze of lemon to taste
- Salt and pepper to taste
- Lemon zest from one lemon
- ½ cup of plain whole fat yogurt
- ¼ cup of chopped parsley
- 1 tablespoon [olive oil](#)
- 1 garlic clove, finely minced
- Lemon zest
- Cracked pepper to taste
- ¼ teaspoon [salt](#)
- ¼ cup of chopped dill

Directions

- Preheat your oven ready to 375°F.
- Toss asparagus with a drizzle of [olive oil](#) .

- Season and place on a parchment -lined sheet pan .

- Place the salmon in the middle of the asparagus and drizzle with olive oil

- Season with salt and pepper, lemon zest.

- Bake in the oven for 20 minutes or more.

- Combine yogurt, olive oil, garlic, lemon zest, salt, dill, and pepper in a small bowl, whisk.

- Serve and enjoy.

Smoked mackerel pate with griddled toast and cress salad

Ingredients

- Extra virgin olive oil
- 400g of smoked mackerel
- 2 sticks of celery
- 200g of light cream cheese
- 6 slices of good bread
- 3 lemons
- 1 small bunch of fresh flat-leaf parsley
- 2 small punnets of cress

Directions

- Break up the mackerel is a blender or food processor slightly.
- Add the cream cheese with bit of parsley leaves, zest and most of the juice of 1 lemon and a few leaves of parsley. Blend until creamy pate. Season.
- Toss the snipped cress, celery leaves, celery sticks, and the remaining parsley leaves.

- Dress with a good squeeze of lemon juice, a splash of extra virgin olive oil, and some salt and pepper.
- Heat a griddle pan till hot.
- Add the bread, in batches, press down with a frying pan to squash against the griddle ridges.
- Toast for 1 minute, turning halfway.
- Serve and enjoy with lemon wedges and herb salad.

Lemony prawn courgette

Ingredients

- 20g of pine nuts
- ½ a fresh red chili
- 1 lemon
- 120 g ripe cherry tomatoes
- 140g of large raw peeled prawns
- Extra virgin olive oil
- 3 medium courgettes
- 1 clove of garlic

Directions

- Preheat the oven to 400°F.
- Place the prawns in a mixing bowl.
- Squeeze in half the juice of lemon.
- Season with sea salt and black pepper.
- Stir well, then leave to one side to mingle flavors.
- Put the cherry tomatoes on a small baking tray, let roast in the hot oven for 7 minutes.
- Place a frying pan over a medium-high heat.

- Add a drizzle of olive oil, then place in the sliced garlic with chili and fry, once golden, add the prawns, let cook for more 3 minutes, turning regularly.
- Place the courgette, cherry tomatoes, and lemon juice in the pan, let cook for 1 minute, tossing often.
- Toast the pine nuts in a dry pan until golden, then lightly crush.
- Divide among plates, scatter over the crushed pine nuts, then drizzle over a little olive oil.
- Serve and enjoy.

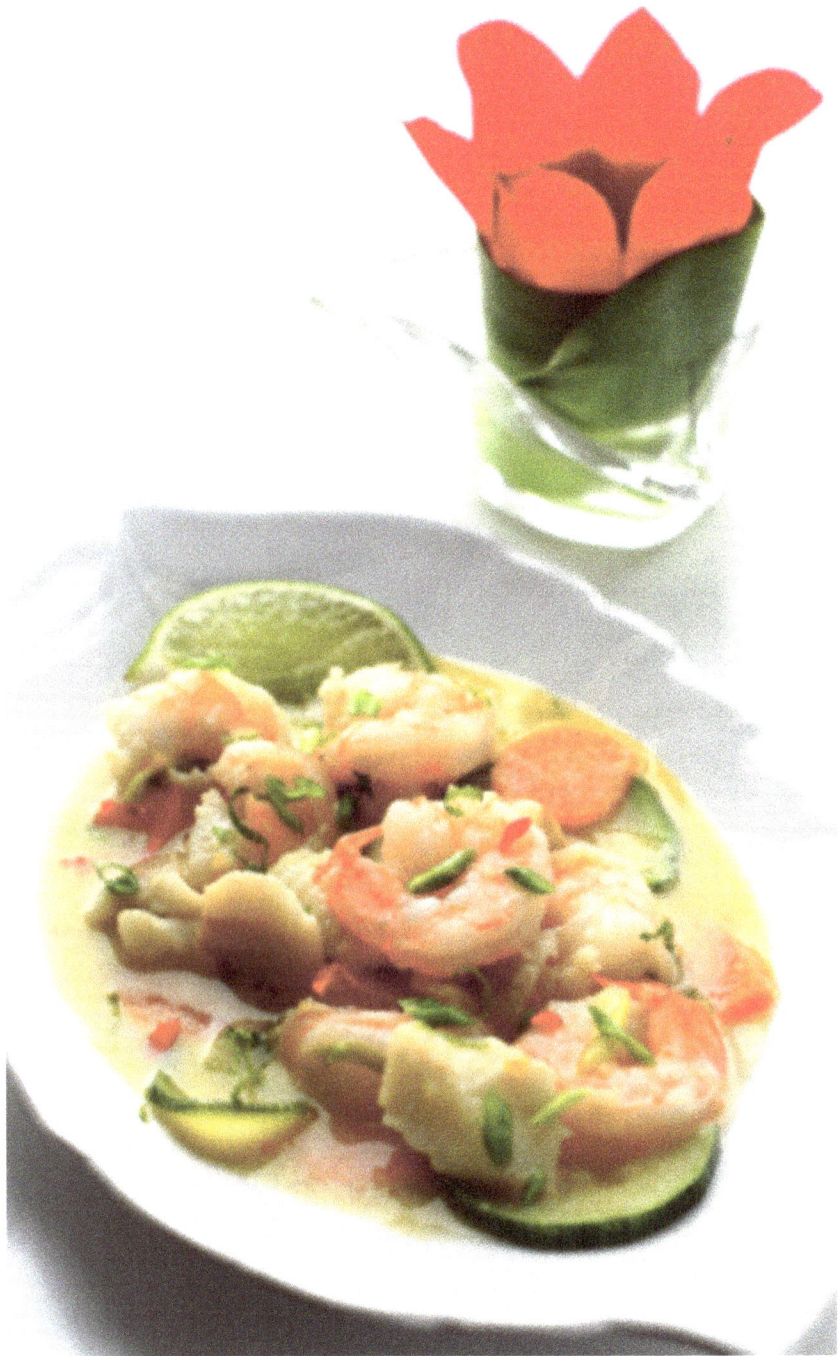

Grilled salmon with herby quinoa

Ingredients

- 4 salmon fillets, skin on
- 160g of ready to eat quinoa
- Extra virgin olive oil
- 2 lemons
- 4 tablespoons of natural yoghurt
- 2 courgettes
- 1 bulb of fennel
- 1 bunch of mixed fresh soft herbs

Directions

- Begin by cooking the quinoa according to the packet Directions.
- Squeeze over the juice of half a lemon.
- Season with a pinch of sea salt and black pepper, set aside.
- Preheat a griddle pan to high.
- Griddle the courgette strips for 2 minutes on each side.
- Place sliced fennel, herb leaves, lemon juice a bowl, stir through the quinoa, season.

- Squeeze the remaining lemon juice into a small bowl, then add the yoghurt with olive oil, stir to combine.
- Season with salt and pepper to taste.
- Season and rub a little olive oil all over the salmon fillets, let cook on the hot griddle for 4 minutes each side.
- Pile the quinoa on a plate and arrange the griddled courgette, lemony fennel on top, with flakes of salmon.
- Serve and enjoy.

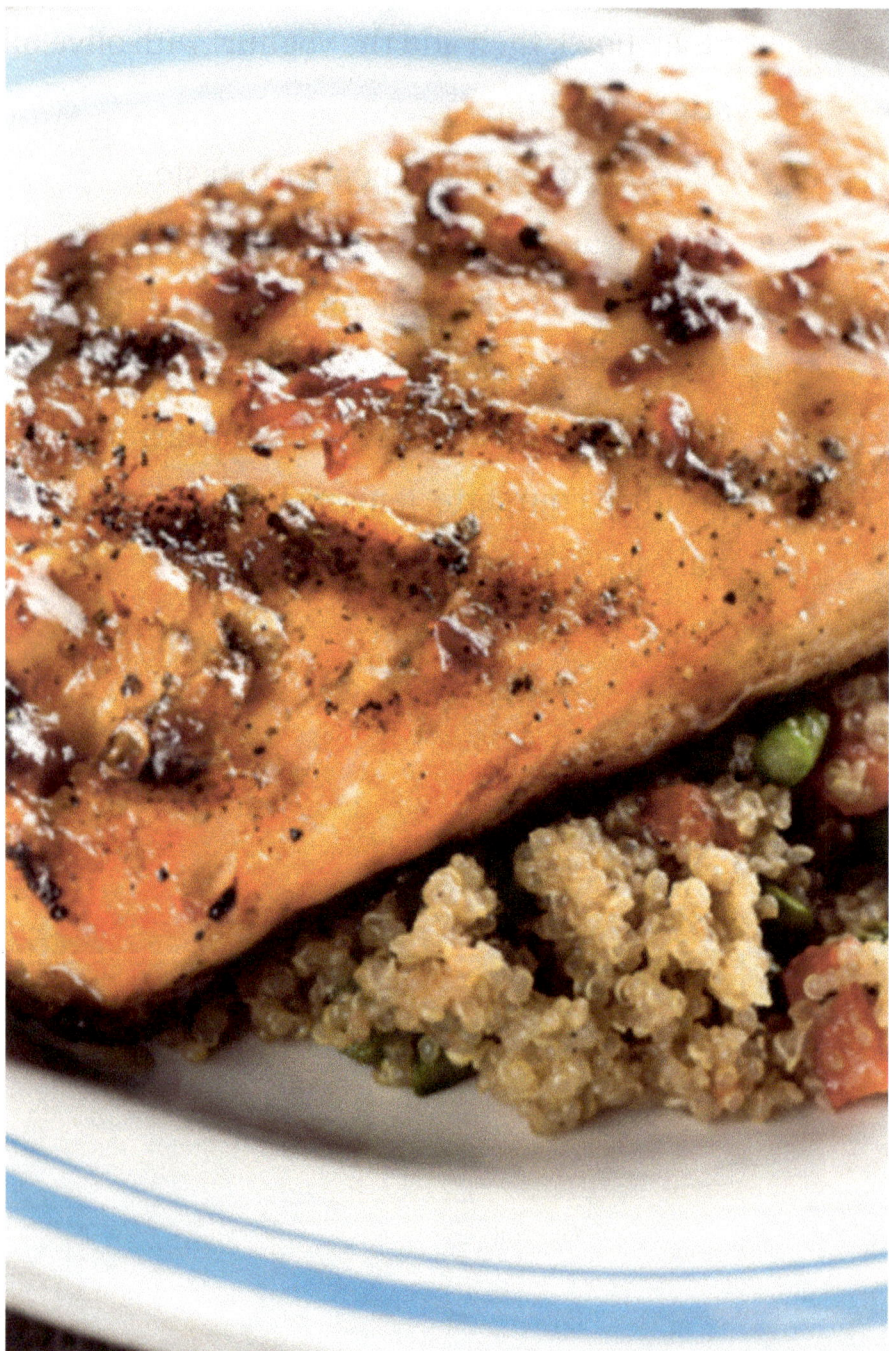

Keralan fish curry

Ingredients

- 1 teaspoon of turmeric
- 6 shallots
- 1 x 400g tin of light coconut milk
- 4 cloves of garlic
- 2.5cm piece of ginger
- 1 tablespoon of chili powder
- 1 x 400g tin of chopped tomatoes
- 1 fresh green chili
- 750g of firm white fish
- A few sprigs of fresh coriander
- Groundnut oil
- 1 teaspoon of mustard seeds
- 20 curry leaves

Directions

- Heat groundnut oil, then add the mustard seeds together with the curry leaves, cook until the seeds begin to pop.

- Add the shallot together with the garlic, ginger, and chili, cook on a medium heat for 5 minutes.
- Mix the chili powder and turmeric with a splash of water, stir into the pan.
- Fry for 1 minute, add the fish together with the coconut milk and tomatoes.
- Season, bring to the boil, let simmer for 20 minutes.
- Scatter the coriander leaves over the dish.
- Serve and enjoy with basmati rice.

Baked sole goujons

Ingredients

- 2 large handfuls of breadcrumbs
- 2 large free-range eggs
- Olive oil
- 50g of plain flour
- 1 tablespoon of sweet smoked paprika
- 450 g lemon sole fillets

Directions

- Preheat the oven to 410°F.
- Cut the fish into finger-width strips.
- Season the flour and place on a plate.
- Crack the eggs into a shallow bowl, lightly beat.
- Mix the paprika with the breadcrumbs on a separate plate.
- Coat the fish goujons with the seasoned flour, dipping them in the eggs, then coating with the breadcrumbs.
- Place them on the oiled tray, let bake until golden.
- Serve and enjoy best with tartare sauce.

Prawn and courgette spaghetti

Ingredients

- 600g of raw peeled prawns
- 2 cloves of garlic
- 3 green courgettes
- 2 fresh red chilies
- ½ lemon
- Parmesan cheese
- 1 bunch of fresh dill
- 2 yellow courgettes
- 500g of dried spaghetti
- 1 large knob of unsalted butter
- Extra virgin olive oil

Directions

- Cook the pasta according to the packet Directions.
- Melt the butter with a splash of oil in a large frying pan on a medium heat.
- Add the courgettes, let cook until slightly browned.

- Add the garlic, chili, and prawns, cook until the prawns are cooked through.
- Remove, squeeze over the lemon juice.
- Drain the pasta, reserving a little cooking water.
- Add the pasta to the frying pan and tossing with the courgettes and prawns.
- Stir in the dill.
- Season, and adjust accordingly.
- Serve and enjoy with a grating of Parmesan.

Green tea roasted salmon

Ingredients

- 1 fresh red chili
- 150g of brown rice
- 1 x 3cm piece of ginger
- 1 x 500g of salmon tail, skin on, scaled, bone in
- Low-salt soy sauce
- ½ a punnet of cress
- 1 green tea bag
- 1 teaspoon of sesame seeds
- Sesame oil
- 1 clove of garlic
- 320g of mixed salad vegetables
- 1 small ripe mango
- 1 lime

Directions

- Preheat your oven to 350°F.
- Then, cook the rice according to package Directions, drain.
- Score the salmon skin at 2cm intervals.

- Season with sea salt and black pepper and the green teabag contents.
- Rub all over with 1 teaspoon of sesame oil, getting well into the cuts.
- Poke a slice of garlic into each cut.
- Let bake for 25 minutes.
- Slice mango flesh into bowl squeezing all the juice, and lime juice with all the vegetables.
- Season with soy sauce.
- Add the chili, then toss with the vegetables and mango.
- Place matchstick ginger, put into a frying pan on a medium heat with 1 teaspoon of sesame oil and seeds.
- Fry until starting to crisp up, tossing regularly.
- Stir in the rice.
- Serve and enjoy with the salmon and rice.

Prawn and papaya salad

Ingredients

- ½ a bunch of fresh basil
- 4 spring onions
- 50g of unsalted peanuts
- Runny honey
- 3 cloves of garlic
- ½ a bunch of fresh coriander
- 400g of peeled prawns
- 1 cucumber
- 4 ripe tomatoes
- 650g of green papaya
- Groundnut oil
- 2 fresh red chilies
- 3 limes
- 3 tablespoons of fish sauce

Directions

- Firstly, toast the peanuts in a large dry frying pan over a medium-high heat
- Transfer to a bowl and set aside.

- Return the frying pan to a medium-high heat with 1 tablespoon of oil and the garlic.
- Fry briefly, then stir in the whole prawns, let fry until turning pink, place in then chopped prawns.
- Cook for 1 minute, stir in the tomatoes, continue to cook for 3 minutes.
- Remove, let cool.
- Add garlic with toasted peanuts into a pestle and mortar, pound to a rough paste.
- Add in lime juice, fish sauce, honey, then mix well.
- Add halved cucumber, shredded green papaya to the dressing.
- Add spring onions, chopped basil leaves, and coriander leaves to the bowl.
- Add the cooled prawn mixture and toss well.
- Roughly chop and scatter over the remaining peanuts.
- Serve and enjoy with lime wedges.

Prawn salad with chili and white cabbage

Ingredients

- Fresh chervil
- Extra virgin olive oil
- 3 handfuls of fresh, raw, small shelled prawns
- 3 lemons, juice of plus the finely grated zest of ½ a lemon
- 1 red chili, seeded and finely sliced
- ½ white cabbage, finely shredded

Directions

- Put the prawns into a shallow dish.
- Squeeze over the juice of 2 lemons, toss slightly to coat, let marinate for 20 minutes. Drain any excess juice.
- Mix the chili with the cabbage.
- Add grated lemon zest with the marinated prawns, a splash of olive oil, and the juice of remaining lemon.
- Toss gently together with the chervil.
- Season with salt and freshly ground black pepper.

- Serve and enjoy.

Roasted cod with pancetta and pea mash

Ingredients

- Extra virgin olive oil
- 4 thick pieces of cod fillet
- ½ a bunch of fresh mint
- 1 small knob of butter
- 8 thin slices of pancetta
- 60g of rocket
- 2 lemons
- 1 splash of milk
- 500g of potatoes
- 300g of frozen garden peas
- ½ a fresh red chili

Directions

- Preheat your oven to 400°F.
- Season the cod with sea salt and black pepper.
- Then, place on an oiled baking tray, lay 2 slices of pancetta over the top of each fillet.
- Place 4 halved lemons on the tray next to the fish.
- Let roast in the preheated oven for 15 minutes.

- Cook the quartered potatoes until soft in boiling salted water.
- Cook the peas according to packet Directions, drain.
- Blend the peas in a food processor.
- Drain the potatoes and mash with butter, hot milk, salt and pepper, whisk the peas and the red chili.
- Put the rocket in a mixing bowl, with the mint leaves, toss together.
- Serve each piece of cod on a dollop of pea and potato mash.
- Enjoy.

Fish in crazy water

Ingredients

- 150g of white wine
- 2 spring onions
- 2 x 350g of whole round fish
- 1 lemon
- ½ a bulb of fennel
- 1 carrot
- 200g of ripe mixed-color cherry tomatoes
- Extra virgin olive oil
- 3 cloves of garlic
- 1 bunch of mixed fresh soft herbs
- ½ of a fresh red chili
- 10 mixed olives
- Olive oil

Directions

- Put a large frying pan on a high heat with 1 tablespoon of olive oil.
- Stir in the onions together with the fennel and carrot.

- After a short while, add the tomatoes, with the garlic, chili, and olives. Toss regularly for 2 minutes.
- Lay the fish on top of the vegetables, then the herbs into the cavities, then pour over the wine.
- Add about 300ml of water, cover, let boil on a high heat for 8 minutes
- Pick the remaining herb leaves, finely grate the lemon zest over them, mix together.
- Uncover the fish, let baste with its juices for 1 minute.
- Remove to a plate, spoon over the vegetables, and juices, drizzle with extra virgin olive oil.
- Scatter over the lemony herbs.
- Serve and enjoy.

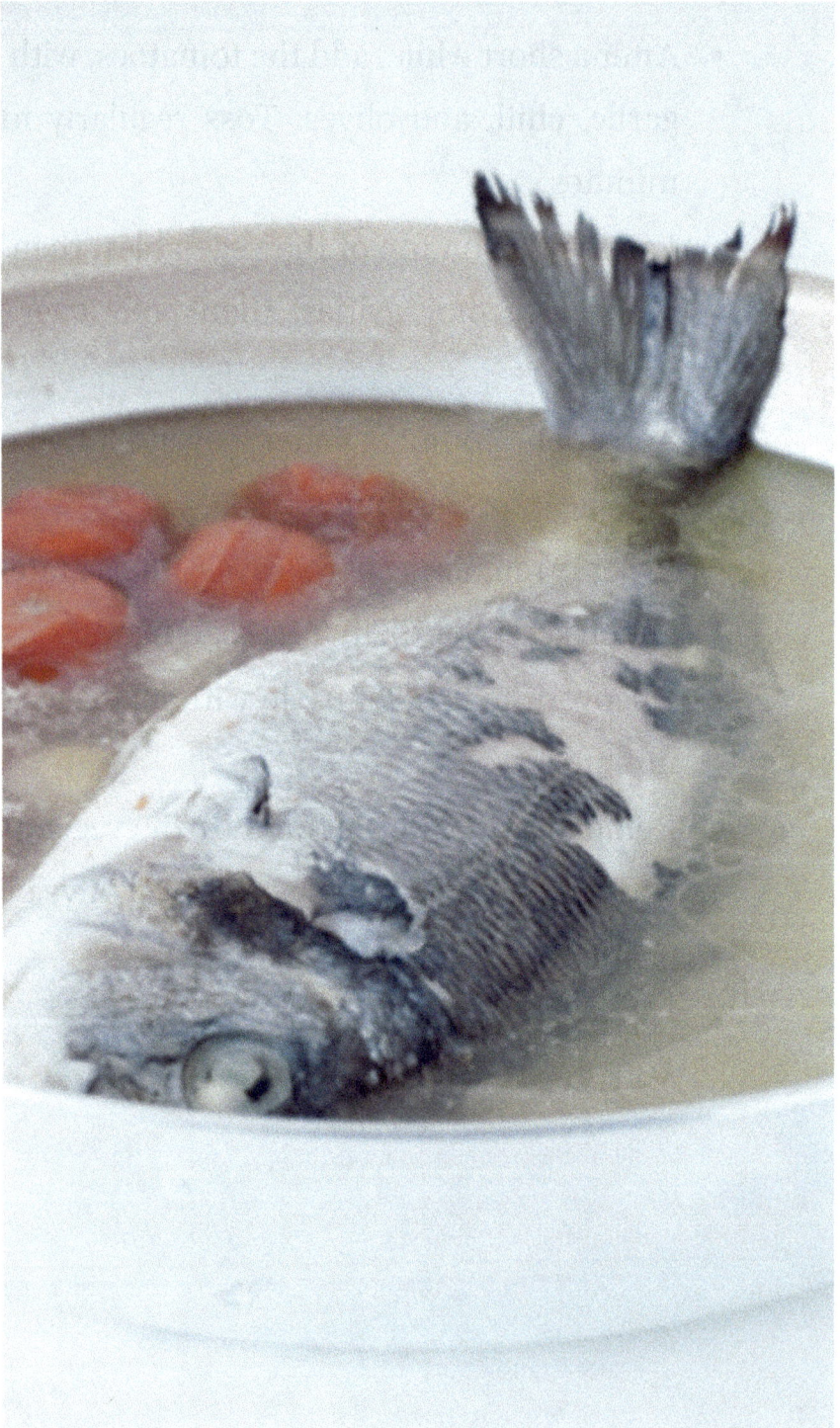

52

Baked tiella rice

Ingredients

- 500g of long-grain rice
- 300g of potatoes
- 750g of mussels
- 400ml of Prosecco
- 1 onion
- 1 clove of garlic
- 1 bunch of fresh flat-leaf parsley
- 2 sticks of celery
- 400g of ripe cherry tomatoes
- 1 courgette
- 60g of Parmesan cheese
- Extra virgin olive oil

Directions

- Preheat the oven to 400°F.
- Place quartered potatoes in an ovenproof earthenware pot.
- Add onion, garlic, tomatoes, parsley, and celery to the pot.

- Place in the Parmesan, and pour in the Prosecco and 8 tablespoons of olive oil.
- Add the rice, season with sea salt and black pepper, then mix.
- Place the mussels into a really hot pan, cover, and steam for 4 minutes until they open.
- Remove the mussel shells.
- Stir the mussels and any juices into the pot, then layer the courgette on top like a lid, grate over the remaining Parmesan.
- Place on a high heat, and as soon as it starts to bubble, transfer to the oven for 45 minutes.
- Let rest, serve and enjoy.

Tuna fettuccine

Ingredients

- 50g of whole almonds
- 1 x 400g tin of cherry tomatoes
- 30g of pecorino cheese
- 4 baby courgettes with flowers
- 1 small onion
- 2 cloves of garlic
- Extra virgin olive oil
- 4 anchovy fillets in oil
- Olive oil
- 1 lemon
- 300g of dried fettuccine
- 300g of yellowfin tuna

Directions

- Lightly toast the almonds in a large frying pan on a medium heat.
- Place into a pestle and mortar.
- Add onion, garlic, anchovies, olive oil to the pan. Fry for 4 minutes, stirring regularly.

- Cook the pasta in a pan of boiling salted water according to package Directions.
- Stir the courgette and tuna into the frying pan.
- Scrunch in the tomatoes with your hands, and lemon juice, let tick away, stirring regularly.
- Finely grate the pecorino. Then, Pound the almonds until fine.
- Once cooked, drag the pasta straight into the frying pan.
- Toss together, then tear in the courgette flowers and toss in the pecorino with most of the almonds.
- Taste and adjust the seasoning.
- Serve and enjoy sprinkled with the remaining almonds.

Jumbo fish fingers

Ingredients

- 30g of Cheddar
- 200g of whole meal bread
- 2kg of salmon
- 2 large free-range eggs
- 100g of plain flour
- Extra virgin olive oil
- 2 teaspoons of sweet smoked paprika

Directions

- Cut the fish into equal portions
- Sprinkle the flour across a plate.
- Then, in a shallow bowl, whisk the eggs together with the paprika and a pinch of sea salt and black pepper.
- Place the bread into a food processor with the cheese, olive oil, sea salt and black pepper, whisk until breadcrumbs form. Place into a baking tray.
- Turn each fish portion in the flour to coat.

- Then, dip in the egg mixture, and later turn it in the breadcrumbs until well coated.
- Transfer to a baking tray lined with greaseproof paper, layering them up between sheets of paper until all of the fish is coated.
- Cook immediately or freeze in the tray.
- To cook, place jumbo fish fingers on the roasting tray, cook in the oven at 400°F for 15 minutes and 20 minutes for fresh and frozen fish respectively.
- Serve and enjoy when the time is up.

Five-spice salmon tacos

Ingredients

- 2 shallots
- 1 tablespoon of white wine vinegar
- 4 x 125g of salmon fillets, skin on
- 1 fresh red chili
- 1 pinch of sugar
- 3 teaspoons of five spice powder
- 4 corn or flour tortillas
- Olive oil
- ½ a bunch of fresh coriander
- ½ a bunch of fresh mint
- 150g of plain yoghurt
- 1 cucumber

Directions

- Start by rubbing the salmon flesh with the five spice, a drizzle of olive oil, and a pinch of sea salt and black pepper.
- Then, heat a frying pan over a medium heat.
- Place the salmon skin-side down in the pan, let cook for 9 minutes.

- Remove shortly after flipping.
- Chop the coriander leaves (reserving a few), and the mint leaves, then combine with the yoghurt.
- Season to taste.
- Place cucumber ribbons, shallots, and chili in a bowl, then sprinkle over the vinegar, sugar, and a pinch of salt, and mix with hands to combine.
- Place a tortilla on each plate and flake over the salmon fillets.
- Add a dollop of yoghurt, minty cucumber, and reserved coriander leaves.
- Roll up and enjoy.

Baked sole goujons

Ingredients

- 50g of plain flour
- 1 tablespoon of sweet smoked paprika
- 2 large free-range eggs
- Olive oil
- 2 large handfuls of breadcrumbs
- 450g of lemon sole fillets

Directions

- Preheat your oven to 420°F.
- Cut the fish into finger-width strips.
- Season the flour and place it on a plate.
- Crack the eggs into a shallow bowl, and beat lightly.
- Mix the paprika with the breadcrumbs on another plate.
- Coat the fish goujons with the seasoned flour, dipping them in the eggs, then coating with the breadcrumbs.
- Place them on the oiled tray and bake for 15 minutes, until golden.

- Serve and enjoy with tartare sauce.

Sesame seared salmon

Ingredients

- 2 x 100 g fillets of salmon
- 4 teaspoons of sesame seeds
- 8cm piece of cucumber
- 2 small carrots
- 1 clove of garlic
- 2 sprigs of fresh coriander
- 2 raw baby beets
- 1 punnet of cress
- 150g of brown rice noodles
- 4 teaspoons tahini
- 1 ripe avocado
- Extra virgin olive oil
- 2 limes
- 1 fresh red chili

Directions

- Cook the noodles according to the packet Directions.
- Drain and toss in a little squeeze of lime juice.

- Carefully slice each of the salmon fillets lengthways into three.
- Scatter the sesame seeds over a board and press one side of the salmon slices into the seeds to form a crust.
- Place a large dry frying pan over a medium heat, and once hot, add the salmon sesame-side down. Leave for 3 minutes.
- Pound the garlic with a pinch of sea salt in a pestle and mortar, then muddle in the tahini, the remaining lime juice, and a splash of water to make a wicked dressing.
- Use a box grater to coarsely grate the cucumber, carrots and beets, keeping them in separate piles and dividing between two plates.
- Snip and divide up the cress, then divide up the noodles.
- Add one half of avocado to each plate.
- Lay the salmon alongside, then finely slice the chili and scatter over with the coriander leaves.
- Toss everything together at the table.

- Serve and enjoy.

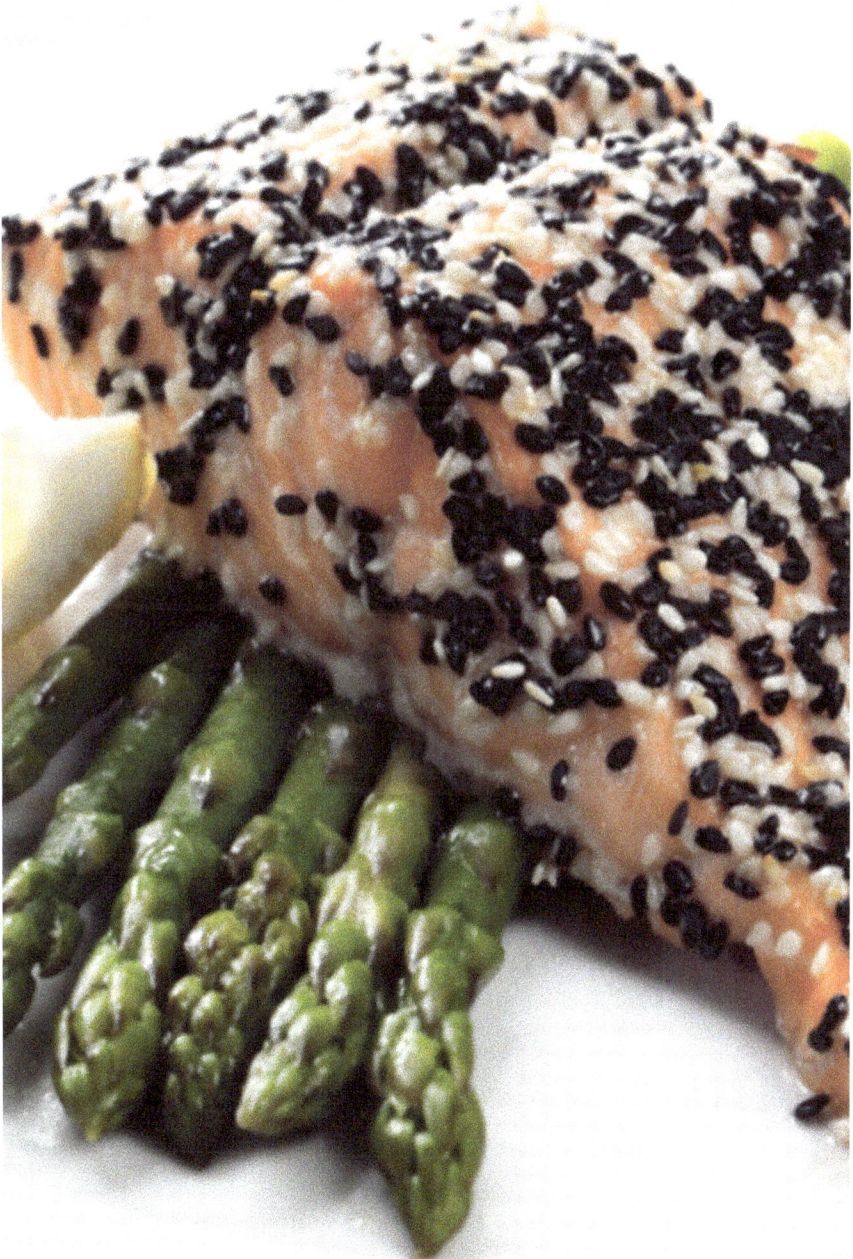

Sicilian fish soup

Ingredients

- ½ lemon
- 1 red onion
- 2 sticks celery
- 1 large handful fresh flat-leaf parsley, chopped
- ½ small bulb fennel
- 2 cloves garlic
- ½ butternut squash, peeled and grated
- 1 red chili, deseeded
- 200g of salmon fillet
- 12 raw peeled prawns or langoustine tails
- 300g of halibut fillet
- 2 tablespoons of olive oil
- 1 glass of dry white wine
- 800g of chopped plum tomatoes
- 500ml of organic fish stock

Directions

- Finely chop the onion, celery, fennel, garlic and chili.
- Then, heat the oil in a large pan.

- Add the onion together with the celery, fennel, garlic, and chili and sweat gently until soft.
- Add the wine, tomatoes or passata, squash, and stock and bring to the boil.
- Cover and simmer gently for 30 minutes.
- Season and gently break up the tomatoes.
- Roughly chop the salmon and halibut and add to the pan.
- Add the prawns or langoustine tails, cover and simmer for 10 minutes.
- Taste the soup and season and adjust.
- Serve and enjoy drizzled with olive oil and sprinkled with the chopped parsley.

Carbonara of smoked mackerel

Ingredient

- 2 sprigs of fresh rosemary
- 320g of dried penne
- 2 large eggs
- 1 lemon
- 40g of Parmesan cheese
- 1 onion
- 1 large courgette
- 100ml of semi-skimmed milk
- 130g of smoked boneless mackerel fillets
- Olive oil

Directions

- Cook the penne in a pan of boiling salted water as instructed on the package.
- Place the onions together with the courgettes into a large frying pan on a medium heat with olive oil.
- Season with a pinch of sea salt and black pepper, stirring occasionally.

- Add the rosemary with the mackerel after 5 minutes, let cook for a further 5 minutes, tossing occasionally.
- Then, whisk the eggs and milk together, then grate in the Parmesan.
- Drain the pasta once ready, reserving some water for later, toss into a mackerel pan.
- Remove the pan briefly, stir in splash of the reserved water to cool it down.
- Quickly pour in the egg mixture, stir until thickened, and evenly coated.
- Serve and enjoy with an extra grating of Parmesan.

Mighty mackerel

Ingredients

- 2 heaped teaspoons of jarred grated horseradish
- 1 heaped teaspoon of ground coriander
- 1 mug of quinoa
- 2 sprigs of fresh rosemary
- ½ a lemon
- A few sprigs of fresh basil
- 800g of ripe mixed-color tomatoes
- 1 fresh red chili
- 2 tablespoons of extra virgin olive oil
- 2 heaped tablespoons of natural yoghurt
- 2 cloves of garlic
- 1 tablespoon of balsamic vinegar
- 4 x 200g of whole mackerel
- Olive oil

Directions

- Place the quinoa, pinch of sea salt, lemon half, and 2 mugs of boiling water into the medium pan, cover, stir frequently.

- Then, score the mackerel on both sides down to the bone on a greaseproof paper.
- Rub all over with salt, black pepper and the ground coriander.
- Place into the large frying pan with bit of olive oil.
- Arrange tomatoes on a large board and sprinkle over with the chili.
- Strip the rosemary leaves over the fish, then add the whole garlic cloves.
- Turn the fish when golden.
- Drain the quinoa when ready, squeeze the lemon juice over it.
- Spoon the quinoa into the center of the tomatoes.
- Drizzle with 2 tablespoons of extra virgin olive oil, balsamic, and a pinch of salt and pepper.
- Then, lay the crispy fish on top.
- Mix the yoghurt with the horseradish
- Serve and enjoy.

Mackerel plaki

Ingredients

- 4 sprigs of fresh flat-leaf parsley
- 8 small whole mackerel
- 3 fresh bay leaves
- 3 teaspoons of extra virgin olive oil
- 2 carrots
- 150ml of dry white wine
- 2 onions
- 4 ripe tomatoes
- 3 cloves of garlic
- 1 lemon

Directions

- Preheat the oven to 350°F.
- Peel and thinly slice the carrots, then peel and slice the onions.
- Roughly chop the tomatoes and finely chop the cloves of garlic.
- Place the fish together with the onion, tomato, carrot, garlic, and bay leaves in a baking dish.

- Season with sea salt and black pepper, then drizzle over the oil.
- Sprinkle the chopped parsley over the fish.
- Squeeze in the lemon juice, then, add the wine and a little water.
- Let bake for 30 minutes or until the sauce has thickened.
- Serve and enjoy with an extra squeeze of lemon.

Pan-cooked asparagus mixed with fish

Ingredients

- 1 small handful of thyme tips
- Olive oil
- Extra virgin olive oil
- 2 small red mullet
- 1 lemon
- 1 royal bream fillet
- 2 small squid
- 4 freshly shelled scallops
- 1 small handful of fennel tops
- 10 medium asparagus spears
- 1 fresh red chili

Directions

- Place a large frying pan to heat with olive oil.
- Score the skin of the fish fillets and season.
- Place the fillets into the pan, skin side down, with the squid tentacles.
- Add the scallops.
- Then, run your knife down one side of each squid to open them out.

- Slightly score the inside in a crisscross fashion.
- Lay in the pan, scored side down.
- Add the asparagus, gently shake the pan.
- Cook briefly, then turn everything over and cook the other side.
- Sprinkle over the thyme tips.
- When the fish and scallops turn golden on the edges, remove the pan.
- Place the squid on a chopping board, slice into pieces, then return to the pan.
- Lay the fish fillets on each plate.
- Toss the asparagus, scallops, and squid with half the chili and a good drizzle of extra virgin olive oil.
- Taste and season accordingly.
- Divide on top of the plated fish.
- Sprinkle with the rest of the chopped chili and the fennel tops.
- Serve and enjoy with extra virgin olive oil.

Peruvian seafood stew with cilantro broth

Ingredients

- 1 green bell pepper
- 6 cloves garlic
- 1 tablespoon of coriander
- 2 teaspoons of cumin
- 2 lbs. seafood
- 4 cups of chicken broth
- 2 tablespoons olive oil
- 3 cups of water
- 4 cups of small diced potatoes
- 1 yellow or white onion
- Juice of 3 limes
- 2 cup of diced carrots
- ½ teaspoon of cracked pepper
- 2 whole bunches of cilantro
- 1 fresh green ancho chili
- 1 teaspoon of kosher salt

Directions

- Heat oil over medium high heat.

- Add onion, let sauté for 3 minutes, stirring often.
- Add ancho chili with bell pepper.
- Add garlic with spices, cook briefly until fragrant.
- Transfer to a blender , set aside.
- In the same pot, add 4 cups of chicken broth and water boil.
- Add the small diced potatoes and carrots, simmer over medium heat for 10 minutes.
- Add two whole bunches of cilantro to the blender , with water, blend until smooth. Keep for later.
- Add all the seafood simmer for 3 minutes.
- Stir in blended cilantro mixture from the blender .
- Season and adjust accordingly.
- Serve and enjoy.

Seared black cod with Meyer lemon risotto and gremolata

Ingredients

- 1 cup of white onion, finely diced
- Salt and pepper
- 1 cup white wine
- 1-pound filet of Black Cod
- 1 garlic clove- finely minced
- 5 cups hot water or stock
- 2 tablespoons of butter or oil
- ¼ teaspoon of white pepper
- 3 Meyer lemons, juice and zest
- ½ cup of chopped Italian parsley
- 2 cups of aborio rice
- ½ cup of olive oil

Directions

- Melt butter over medium heat.
- Add onions, sauté until tender.
- Add rice, sauté for 5 minutes, stirring often.
- Add wine over medium-low and stir to absorb.

- Add ½ cup of hot water and stir to absorb for 20 minutes over low heat.
- Season with <u>salt</u> , <u>white pepper</u> , and zest.
- Combine parsley, lemon juice, olive oil, garlic and salt.
- Heat <u>olive oil</u> over medium high heat.
- Pat dry fish and season.
- Place skin side down in the skillet and sear.
- Continue searing over low heat for 5 minutes, until skin is crisp.
- Serve and enjoy with roasted asparagus.

Grilled fish tacos with cilantro lime cabbage slaw

Ingredients

- ½ cup chopped cilantro
- ½ of a jalapeño
- 1 ½ teaspoon of chili powder
- ¼ cup fresh lime juice
- 1 teaspoon of cumin
- 2 tablespoon of olive oil
- 1 teaspoon of coriander
- 1 teaspoon of granulated garlic
- ½ teaspoon of sugar
- 2 lbs. of grill able white fish
- ¼ teaspoon of chipotle powder
- 3/4 teaspoon of kosher salt
- 1 pound of thinly sliced or shredded cabbage
- ¼ cup of thinly sliced red onion

Directions

- Preheat your grill ready to medium heat.
- Place the shredded cabbage in a medium bowl. Toss with the salt .

- Add onions together with cilantro, lime juice, jalapeño, olive oil and toss well.
- Grill each side briefly, letting grill marks develop, flip to grill the other side.
- Grill the tortillas, brush with olive oi
- Serve and enjoy.

Quick and easy salmon cakes

Ingredients

- Salt and pepper
- 1 egg
- 2 tablespoons sour cream
- 3 tablespoon of mayo
- 1 teaspoon of lemon juice
- 2 tablespoons fresh dill
- Squeeze of lemon
- ½ teaspoon of garlic powder
- 1 can of salmon
- ⅓ cup of toasted bread crumbs
- 2 scallions, sliced
- Olive oil for searing

Directions

- Mix all ingredients together in a medium bowl. Let settle for 10 minutes.
- Divide mixture into 2 larger cakes pressing together with your hands.
- Heat oil in a skillet over medium heat.

- Sear the salmon cakes for 5 minutes on each side until golden.
- Serve with the quick creamy sauce.
- Enjoy.

Balinese fish and potato curry

Ingredients

- Sambal oelek
- 12 ounces of while fish
- 1 tablespoon of fresh turmeric
- 2 x 5 inch stocks lemongrass
- 1 cup of peas
- 3 garlic cloves
- 1 tablespoon of fish sauce
- 1 jalapeno
- 5 kefir lime leaves
- 2 tablespoons of coconut oil
- 2 cups of water
- 10 ounces of baby potatoes
- 2 tablespoons of thinly sliced ginger
- 1 can of coconut milk
- ½ teaspoon of salt
- 1 shallot rough chopped
- 1 lime- juice

Directions

- Cook rice as instructed on the package.

- Place the thinly sliced ginger together with the lemongrass, shallot, and turmeric in the food processor .
- Add the jalapeño, garlic, and lime leaves. Pulse to foam.
- Heat coconut oil over medium high heat.
- Add the paste and stir constantly for 4 minutes.
- Add and boil 2 cups of water.
- Add potatoes, cover let simmer for 15 minutes.
- Add coconut milk with salt , fish sauce and lime juice
- Taste, and adjust accordingly.
- Place the fish into the coconut sauce and simmer for 5 minutes.
- Place in the spring peas cook briefly.
- Serve and enjoy with lime wedges.

Pasty's garlic and chili prawns

Ingredients

- ½ teaspoon of smoked paprika
- 1 lemon
- 3 cloves of garlic
- 1 fresh red chili
- 8 large raw shell-on king prawns
- Sprigs of fresh flat-leaf parsley
- 50ml of olive oil

Directions

- Drizzle oil into a shallow heatproof terracotta dish over a medium-high heat.
- Add garlic with chili and fry briefly.
- Stir in the paprika.
- Add the prawns and parsley, fry for 2 minutes on each side.
- Squeeze half the lemon juice into the dish.
- Remove and sprinkle over the remaining parsley and a pinch of sea salt.
- Serve and enjoy with lemon wedges.

Paella

Ingredients

- 500g of paella rice
- 6 free-range chicken thighs
- 1 heaped teaspoon of smoked paprika
- 500g of mussel
- olive oil
- 100g of quality chorizo
- 10 large raw shell-on king prawns
- 1 onion
- 1 lemon
- 4 cloves of garlic
- Plain flour
- ½ a bunch of fresh flat-leaf parsley
- 6 rashers of higher-welfare pancetta
- 2 liters of organic chicken stock
- 2 handfuls of fresh or frozen peas
- 2 large pinches of saffron
- 2 small squid

Directions

- Preheat the oven to 375°F.

- Heat a splash of oil over medium heat, fry the chicken until golden brown.
- Bake for 20 minutes.
- Return the pan to heat, add chorizo and pancetta, fry until browned.
- Add the onion together with the garlic and parsley stalks, cook until soft.
- Heat and infuse the chicken stock with the saffron.
- Add the smoked paprika, rice and infused stock to the pan, let cook for around 20 minutes on low heat.
- Add the remaining stock, peas, prawns, and the mussels, let cook for 10 minutes.
- Add the cooked chicken, sprinkle over the chopped parsley.
- Serve and enjoy with wedges.

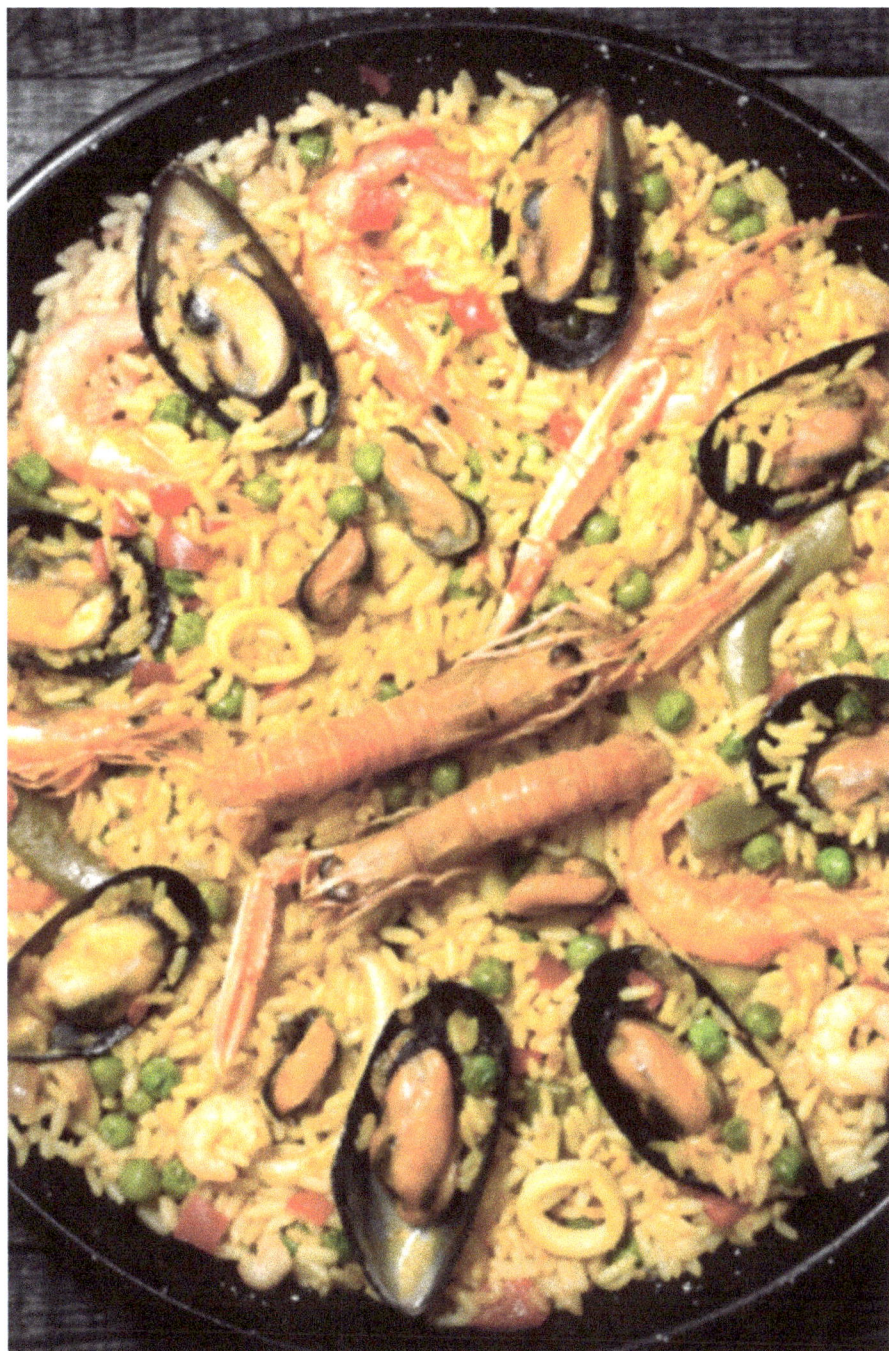

Retro crab cocktail

Ingredients

- 1 tablespoon of tomato ketchup
- ¼ of a cucumber
- Cayenne pepper
- 1 lemon
- 1 ripe avocado
- 6 radishes
- 300g of cooked white crab meat
- 1 punnet of cress
- 1 punnet of micro herbs
- ½ of an iceberg lettuce
- 3 tablespoons of mayonnaise
- 1 teaspoon of Worcestershire sauce

Directions

- Mix the mayo, ketchup, and Worcestershire sauce in a bowl.
- Add lemon juice with brandy.
- Season with sea salt and black pepper.
- Mix the crabmeat with the mayo

- Divide the crab between the plates and drizzle over a little Marie Rose sauce.
- Serve and enjoy.

Seared tuna steak

Ingredients

- 1 handful of fresh coriander
- 1 small dried red chili
- Tuna steaks
- 1 tablespoon of coriander seeds
- 1 lemon
- ½ clove of garlic
- 1 handful of fresh basil
- Olive oil

Directions

- Combine the garlic, herb leaves, olive oil, and lemon juice, mix in a mortar.
- Season with salt and pepper.
- Lay out the tuna steaks on a tray, season both sides, rub with the herb mixture.
- Place in the tuna, toasts and fry for 60 seconds on each side.
- Serve and enjoy with potatoes.

Honeymoon spaghetti

Ingredients

- 1 large free-range egg
- 5 cloves of garlic
- 1 fresh red chili
- 1 fresh red chili
- 450g of mussels
- 1.5kg of crab
- 100g of squid
- 2 x 400g tins of plum tomatoes
- 30g of unsalted butter
- 200g of raw shell-off tiger prawns
- 450g of dried spaghetti
- 1 bunch of flat-leaf parsley
- 1 bunch of marjoram
- 3 cloves of garlic

Directions

- Preheat the oven to 350°F.
- Boil crab for 15 minutes, let cool.
- Remove the meat, flake into small pieces.
- Combine pounded shells with chopped garlic.

- Drizzle with olive oil over a medium heat and fry.
- Add the broken tomatoes with water, simmer for 1 hour.
- Sieve, season with sea salt and black pepper.
- Cook the spaghetti as instructed on the package. Drain.
- Melt the butter with olive oil. Add garlic and chili to the pan, fry. S
- Raise the heat, then mussel prawns let cook for 2 minutes.
- Remove from the heat, discard unopened mussels.
- Add tomato sauce, pasta parsley, marjoram leaves, and crab, mix.
- Place the seafood mixture in the center of a baking tray, beat the egg.
- Use it to brush the edges, seal and cook for 10 minutes.
- Serve and enjoy.

Seafood risotto

Ingredients

- ½ a bunch of fresh rosemary
- Olive oil
- 6 raw langoustines
- 1.6 liters quality fish stock
- 300g of mussels, scrubbed
- Extra virgin olive oil
- 400g of risotto rice
- 500g of clams, scrubbed
- 2 cloves of garlic
- 4 medium squid
- 300g of cooked white crab meat
- 1 knob of butter
- 1 pinch of saffron
- 400g of mixed cherry tomatoes
- 1 large onion
- 1 heart of celery
- 1 bulb of fennel
- ½ a glass of white wine
- 30g of Parmesan cheese

Directions

- Preheat the oven to 325°F.
- Tip tomatoes into a medium roasting tray.
- Combine garlic, rosemary leaves, tomatoes, olive oil and toss to coat and space them out in a single layer.
- Let roast for 40 minutes
- Put the saffron in a small bowl, cover with 50ml of freshly boiled water, infuse.
- Place onion, celery, fennel in a pan with oil over a medium heat, let cook for 15 minutes, stir in the rice, toast for 2 minutes.
- Pour in the wine, and stir until absorbed.
- Add a ladleful of stock, let it be fully absorbed.
- Add the saffron and its soaking liquid, stir in the mussels with clams.
- Beat in the butter, Parmesan, season.
- Dot over the roasted tomatoes and herbs.
- Serve and enjoy.

Grilled squid salad

Ingredients

- ½ a bunch of fresh mint
- 2 tablespoons of baby capers in brine
- 500g of large ripe tomatoes
- 2 lemons
- Extra virgin olive oil
- 4 large squid
- 1 clove of garlic
- 30g of shelled unsalted pistachios
- 1 fresh red chili
- 4 anchovy fillets in oil

Directions

- Combine garlic, chili, anchovies, pistachios, capers, and mint leaves in a mixing bowl. Mix well.
- Add the tubes, from largest to smallest. Cook each piece for about 1 minute per side.
- As each piece is done, use tongs to dunk it straight into the salsa, turning and coating it in flavor.

- Slice the tomatoes and lay over a serving platter.
- Slice the squid tubes, pull the tentacles apart, then arrange on top of the tomatoes.
- Serve and enjoy.

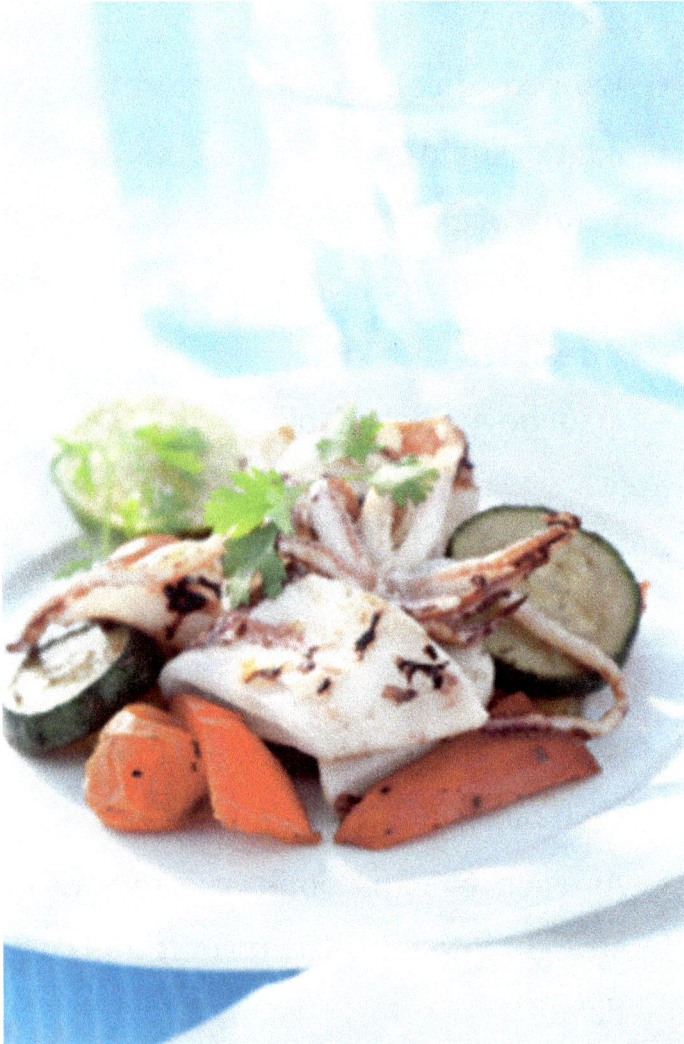

Stuffed braised squid

Ingredients

- 25g of baby capers in brine
- 4 medium squid
- 300g of dried spaghetti
- 1 x 680g jar of passata
- 100g of coarse stale breadcrumbs
- 2 sprigs of fresh basil
- Olive oil
- 15g of pecorino
- 1 clove of garlic
- ½ a bunch of fresh flat-leaf parsley
- 1 red onion
- 1 large free-range egg
- 10 ripe cherry tomatoes

Directions

- Place half the capers in a bowl with the breadcrumbs, garlic, pecorino, egg, olive oil and water, mix.
- Combine onions, tomatoes, add to pan with passata and let Simmer on a low heat.

- Fill squid tubes with breadcrumb mixture seal with toothpick.
- Stir the remaining capers into the sauce, with stuffed squid and tentacles.
- Simmer on a low heat for 25 minutes, or until tender.
- cook the pasta according to the packet Directions.
- Transfer the squid to board. Arrange.
- Serve and enjoy.

Prawn and tuna linguine

Ingredients

- 150g of dried linguine
- 4 large raw shell-on prawns
- Olive oil
- 2 small onions
- 1 cinnamon stick
- ½ a bunch of fresh flat-leaf parsley
- 1 good pinch of saffron
- 200g of yellowfin tuna
- 4 tablespoons white wine vinegar
- 2 anchovy fillets in oil
- 50g of shelled unsalted pistachios
- Pecorino or Parmesan cheese rind

Directions

- Over medium heat, place onions, prawn heads, olive oil, and cinnamon in a pan.
- Add anchovies once sizzling. Drain, toss.
- Cook for 20 minutes when covered as you stir occasionally.

- Cook the pasta according to the packet Directions.
- Gently squash each prawn head so all the tasty juices spill out into the pan.
- Stir in half the parsley, prawns, tuna, and saffron vinegar mixture.
- Drag the pasta straight into the pan, letting a little starchy cooking water go with it.
- Toss for 2 minutes.
- Season accordingly.
- Serve and enjoy.

Smoked salmon pate

Ingredients

- 2 lemons
- 150g of cooked peeled prawns
- 150g of quality smoked salmon
- 1 celery heart
- ½ a bunch of fresh dill
- 150g of white crabmeat
- 1 fresh red chili
- 1 loaf of sourdough bread
- 280g of cream cheese
- 25g of salmon caviar
- 1 lemon
- Extra virgin olive oil
- Cayenne pepper
- 1 small red onion

Directions

- Place the prawns with smoked fish in a bowl with the crabmeat, grated zest, cream cheese, caviar, and black pepper mix well.
- Spoon into a dish and smooth out evenly.

- Place into the fridge until needed.
- Combine red onion, chili, celery, leaves, dill, and lemon wedges and refrigerate overnight.
- Slice and toast the bread.
- Cut a crisscross pattern into the top of the pâté.
- Drizzle with a little oil and sprinkle with a pinch of cayenne.
- Serve and enjoy.

Chipotle fried fish and clementine bites

Ingredients

- 75g of plain yoghurt
- 400g of white fish fillets
- 2 limes
- 1 teaspoon dried chipotle flakes
- 2 clementine
- 1 liter of vegetable oil
- ½ of a clementine
- 1 teaspoon ground coriander
- ½ a bunch of fresh coriander
- 150g of corn flour
- 1 small clove of garlic
- 150ml of milk

Directions

- Season the chopped fish with sea salt and black pepper, squeeze over the juice of 1 lime. keep aside for 10 minutes.
- Stir coriander leaves through the yoghurt in a small bowl.
- Add garlic and zest of the clementine.

- In a shallow dish combine ground coriander, corn flour and a pinch of salt, mix well.
- Pour the milk into a separate bowl.
- Heat olive oil
- Pat the fish and clementine slices coat with corn flour, dip briefly in the milk.
- Coat again and shake off any excess.
- Deep fry the fish and clementine for 3 minutes.
- Drain any excess oil, scatter with salt, chipotle and the reserved coriander.
- Serve and enjoy immediately.

Crispy Mediterranean Sea base

Ingredients

- 1 lime
- 2 x 300g of whole sea bass
- 4 spring onions
- 2 tablespoons of red curry paste
- ½ a bunch of fresh coriander

Directions

- Place a large non-stick frying pan on a medium temperature.
- Place onions in ice cold water to crisp.
- Pack the coriander stalks into the cavities
- Season with sea salt and black pepper, place in the hot pan with olive oil.
- Let cook for 4 minutes per side.
- Drain and shake off the spring onions and coriander.
- Sit the sea bass on top, spooning over any spicy oil from the pan.
- Serve and enjoy.

Smoked salmon, prawns and Miami cocktail sauce

Ingredients

- 2 tablespoons of chili sauce
- 2cm of piece of ginger
- Sprigs of fresh coriander
- 4 tablespoons of tomato ketchup
- 3 baby gem lettuces
- 300g of smoked salmon
- 24 large cooked peeled prawns
- 1 lime
- 1 teaspoon of English mustard
- ½ a large clove of garlic
- Extra virgin olive oil
- 1 spring onion
- 4 tablespoons of free-range mayonnaise

Directions

- Combine garlic, spring onion, coriander leaves, mayonnaise, tomato ketchup, chili, ginger, and mustard. Mix.
- Place in the fridge for 1 hour.

- Drape the lettuce over the smoked salmon, organize the prawns on top.
- Dress the lettuce and seafood with the cocktail sauce.
- Cut the lime into wedges and squeeze a little juice over each plate.
- Serve and enjoy with black pepper.

Roasted scallops with pancetta and hazelnuts

Ingredients

- 150g of hazelnuts
- 4 scallops in the half shell
- 1 small onion
- 1 sprig of fresh tarragon
- 80g of pancetta
- 2 cloves of garlic
- Olive oil

Directions

- Preheat the oven to 350°F.
- Place a frying pan over a medium heat and drizzle with a little oil.
- Add the pancetta, garlic, and onion let fry until golden.
- Toast and roughly chop the hazelnuts with tarragon, place on one side.
- Divide the pancetta mixture between the scallops, pouring any juices from the pan over the top.

- Bake in the preheated oven 7 minutes, or until the flesh is no longer translucent.
- Sprinkle the chopped hazelnuts over the scallops
- Serve and enjoy with tarragon leaves.

www.ingramcontent.com/pod-product-compliance
Lightning Source LLC
Chambersburg PA
CBHW050752030426
42336CB00012B/1778